CANCER?
We've Got This!

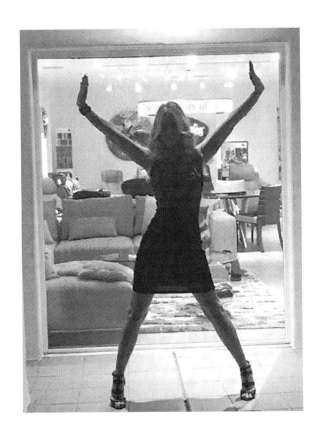

Juliet Mitchell

First Edition

For information about wholesale or bookstore orders,
please contact: Pure Girl in a Toxic World
www.puregirlinatoxicworld.com

Manufactured in the USA
ISBN-10: 0-692-93118-X
ISBN-13: 978-0-692-93118-9

DISCLAIMER

Please note: Within the pages of this book, the information gathered and written has been carefully compiled in order to help readers make choices about their health. However, it should not be considered as a substitute for the advice or treatment offered by licensed doctors and healthcare providers. Juliet is not a doctor, nor a nutritionist.

The author has meticulously gathered data – both from reputable and nationally-recognized sources – in order to provide the most accurate and detailed information. However, neither the author or publisher will be held responsible for any adverse outcomes that may result if a person relies solely on the contents of this book, as well as any errors or omissions herewith.

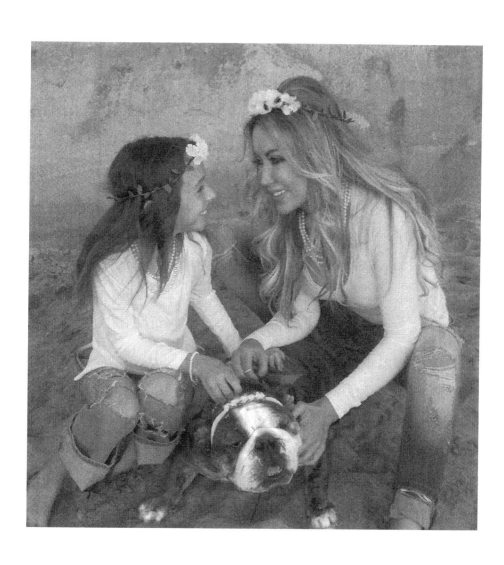

DEDICATION

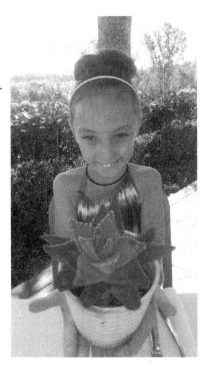

For my loving daughter Katie, you are my world. You gave me the reason to fight the fight of cancer. Without your love, laughter, innocence, smile and your beautiful, sweet, caring heart, I would not have had the strength to find a better life for me and you. I love you to all the universes and back. My pumpkin and my pop chewy princess. I will love you until eternity.

Love, Mommy

To God, thank you for all the people you sent my way to take care of me when I could not take care of myself. I am grateful for your still, loving voice cheering me on. Telling me that I will live and that all I need to do is to trust in you." Your life is God's gift to you, what you do with it is your gift to god". God thank you for the 2nd gift of life. The do over. I hope you love my gift back to you.

Love, Juliet

5

TABLE OF CONTENTS

FOREWORD
By Dr. Afshin Bahador
9

INTRODUCTION
By Juliet Mitchell
13

CHAPTER ONE
My Story
17

CHAPTER TWO
What I Do
43

CHAPTER THREE
If You Are Currently Going Through Chemo & Radiation
61

CHAPTER FOUR
Do's
67

CHAPTER FIVE
Don'ts
87

CONCLUSION
Now It's Your Turn
105

ABOUT THE AUTHOR
Juliet Mitchell
107

TESTIMONIALS
People I've Helped
111

ACKNOWLEDGEMENTS
People Who've Helped Me
114

REFERENCES
Sources for Research in this Book
120

NOTE TAKING
A Place to Jot Down Your Favorite Do's & Don'ts
123

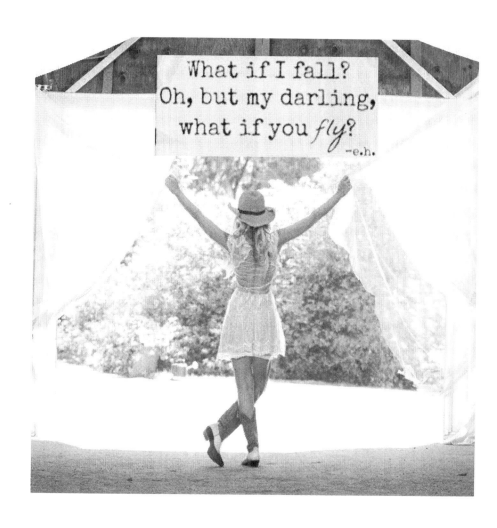

FOREWORD

By Dr. Afshin Bahador

"Let food be thy medicine and medicine be thy food."

--HIPPOCRATES

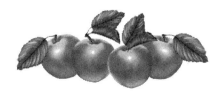

I first had the pleasure of meeting Juliet Mitchell under less-than-desirable circumstances. As a doctor, it is never easy to tell patients about a diagnosis that is unexpected and unfavorable. Having to explain; "You have ovarian cancer," and the subsequent steps needed to handle it is a bit like walking on eggshells. Some patients crack, while others hold up to the news with resilience. Juliet was somewhere in between, but what she did after the news was what impressed me the most about her.

Rather than lying down and taking it, Juliet rose to the occasion like a soldier. Once the initial shock wore off, she diligently went home and dug deep within herself to make her health the top priority in her life. She knew that she had a fierce battle to win, and that is exactly what she did.

In all my years of practicing medicine, I have never seen a more curious patient. Not only did she absorb and take to heart every piece of advice offered, Juliet researched the how's, why's, and the do's and don'ts of this ugly disease most thoroughly. She enrolled in a program at Harvard University to study food, nutrition, and wellbeing. She read every book she could get her hands on, even those I recommended. She studied successful outcomes of cancer survivors and she listened to every shred of advice given.

As a doctor, I do practice what I preach. I believe in the power of organic living and have seen the positive turns it can take in the lives of my patients and within my own family. Juliet took these examples and turned cancer on its heels; transforming her life from one of despair into empowerment. Juliet was on board with this holistic approach, which included a whole food, all-organic method; combined with natural supplements, coffee enemas and plant-based, Vegan diet. Because she was already fit, Juliet was ahead of the game compared to other people. However, this is not why I think she was so successful.

The primary reason I believe Juliet was able to beat cancer so effectively was because of her mindset. Her overwhelming response was one of an Olympic champion; one who was not to be defeated. Having a positive attitude and state of being was the #1 reason she won the battle. The mind is your most powerful asset.

Aside from adopting a holistic, all-natural and organic approach, finding ways to relieve stress is critical to healing. Meditation, exercise, and happiness are among the 'must-have's' for favorable outcomes.

Change can be difficult, and for some, it may take baby steps each day to fully embrace them. For others – like

Juliet Mitchell – they may wholeheartedly commit with gladiator-like prowess. The first change you should make today, upon reading this book, is to find more ways to bring joy, love and positive energy to your life. By doing so, you will begin to naturally adapt and embrace the healthiness you deserve.

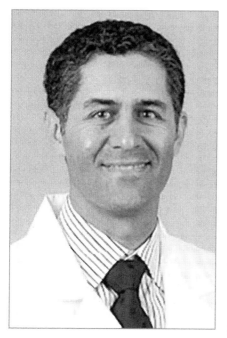

As the saying goes, "Laughter is the best medicine." You could revise that saying by replacing '*laughter*' with '*happiness*'. On that note, I am pleased and humbled to have the opportunity to introduce you to Juliet Mitchell. She is a shining star amidst a grim topic of cancer. Hopefully by the time you finish this book, you will be inspired to follow in her footsteps and take much of the knowledge and research here and apply them to your own life. Start today, and you'll come to admire Juliet as much as I do.

INTRODUCTION

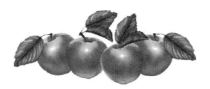

Health is the key to happiness. Just as the saying goes that you cannot buy happiness, well, you can't really buy good health, either. To some extent, having good health can depend upon whether or not you have health insurance, vs. not having any insurance at all. However, even people such as Steve Jobs – who could afford the very best healthcare in the world – could not beat the cancer that eventually killed him.

The reason I wrote this book is because of the lack of books or materials I could find when I was diagnosed with cancer, at least not any that were not several hundred pages long, or with dozens of medical terms that most people don't understand. What I really wanted was for someone credible to tell me specific things that I should do and/or not do. I wanted something simply put – in layman's terms – and that would not require weeks or months to read. Would you believe that I could not find one book that offered this?

So, I did my own research.

When you first hear the words, "Sorry, but you have cancer," it seems shocking and unbelievable. Your brain automatically questions how this could be possible, especially at the young age of 46. It feels as though you are living in a bad nightmare. I was totally overwhelmed with emotions and thoughts of fear. I had millions of thoughts and questions like:

- ➢ "How am I going to handle this?"
- ➢ "Oh my goodness, what about my family and child?"
- ➢ "Where's the money for treatment going to come from?"
- ➢ "Am I going to die?"

On top of all of these unknowns, I wondered how I was going to keep everything in life going at the same time. Kids, work, and domestic responsibilities don't stop just because you get whammed with a thing like cancer. However, deep inside of me there was a little voice I like to call my 'inner child'. It guided me to find ways to help myself and to learn how to bring my body back to good health.

I started by evaluating my lifestyle to learn if there were any factors that may have contributed to this cancer diagnosis. Like a great detective, I wanted to get to the bottom of this mystery. That's where my journey began.

As a result, I was a woman on a mission to beat this cancer. I had an insatiable appetite to learn anything and everything I could get my hands on about cancer. However, I had a hard time focusing, reading, and absorbing those 300-page books about cancer and I could not find any simple reads, except for a handful of pamphlets.

What you are now holding in your hands is literally four years of studying and compiling every shred of information I could find about cancer and being healthy. I took the best things that worked for me and also lifestyle changes that were made to write this book. By sharing what I've learned in an uncomplicated book, my goal is to help other people who have been recently diagnosed with cancer, or even people who want to take a proactive approach in order to decrease their odds of getting it.

While there are no guarantees in life – even for me – I have found the things within the pages of this book to be successful in decreasing my odds of cancer reoccuring. There are 50 Do's and 50 Don'ts, but there are so many more I could have added. I feel that these are the most relevant, but I will encourage you to follow me on puregirlinatoxicworld.com, as well as my Facebook page and Instagram if you want to continue learning updated tips after reading this book.

I keep having to remind myself that this is supposed to be a basic, easy read, and the challenge was in narrowing down the material to make it simple for you, the reader. At the very least, I hope that the information given increases your odds of survival.

Chapter One

My Story

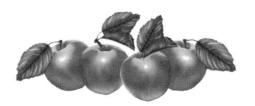

Today is the first day of the rest of your life. I know, you've heard that one before and if you've been diagnosed with cancer, it can feel like a sort of gloomy statement, but only if you take it that way. The rest of your life can be absolutely AWESOME and AMAZING. In fact, I know it's going to be! The information I'm going to share with you is more than a pick-me-up, consider it a lifesaver, but not the fruity, hard candy kind.

If you are just picking up this book up for the first time, whether curiously or fearfully, well... fear not. Imagine that you are just a passenger in my car. I'm going to drive for a while and take you on a ride. While we travel, I'm going to share all the knowledge I have acquired about this difficult topic.

CANCER, it's like the ugliest subject to discuss, isn't it? Nobody ever really likes to talk about cancer. It kills people we love. It is still unsolvable by scientists and researchers, at least for now. There are thousands of pamphlets, books, documentaries, videos and over 644 million websites related to cancer.

However, you don't need any of these. All you need is exactly what you are holding in your hands right now. Yes, my book. I have completed the hard work for you.

I was there once, where you are right now; trying to wade through the oceans worth of information. It was overwhelming. Astoundingly, there was not one, single source in which I could find simple answers to my questions about cancer. I didn't want to read the huge, ginormous textbooks that were 400 pages long. So, I did what any modern woman does these days. I dug. I researched. I Googled until my eyes turned googly-eyed. Yet, there was still never one specific place to find the answers to my questions about cancer.

Now that you are in the passenger seat of my car, buckle up. By the end of this short read, I hope to enlighten you and empower you. I will even pull over and let you take the wheel. My goal for this book is to put you in the driver's seat of your own fate. Yes, cancer sucks, but you can *take back your power*; instead of giving it to cancer.

Welcome! I'm sure we will become fast friends. We already have a few things in common. First, let me tell you about my story.

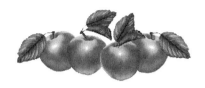

It was July of 2013. While attending my niece's First Holy Communion party, I ran into one of my sister's friends, Lisa. I like to call her the woman that saved my life. We were chatting, just as women do.

"You know Lisa, for some reason I feel like I'm not really getting a good quality sleep like I used to. Plus, I am a bit more bloated than normal," I told her.

"How old are you now, Juliet?"

"I'm 46."

"You might be premenopausal."

"Oh wow!" I exclaimed, a little stunned. "I didn't even think of that one."

"You should go see your OB-GYN, Juliet. She can get you on some hormones that will make you feel a whole lot better," she suggested.

"I'll consider that. Thanks for bringing it to my attention," I said. However, I was busy after the party and kind of blew it off, at least for the time being.

A few days passed. For some odd reason, Lisa's advice kept ringing in my ear. Normally, I would never have taken the suggestion of going to see a doctor just for bloating or abnormal sleep patterns. After all, these were just common symptoms that we all endure from time to time. I come from a tough family; the kind that doesn't show a lot of emotions. We certainly never complain about any problems or illnesses that we are feeling. We put on the 'stiff' upper lip and march on.

On this day, something was different. I sensed an internal nudge within me and felt compelled to make the call. Looking back upon it now, it was God's voice sending a telephone call to me. At any rate, I set up an appointment with my OB-GYN and walked into the office a few days thereafter.

After some idle chit-chat and general inquisitions, my gynecologist agreed that my symptoms sounded like hormone fluctuations. "Let me write you a prescription for estrogen and progesterone," she said, handing me a small slip of paper. "On second thought, let me just make sure that everything is okay first. Juliet, I want you to have an ultrasound. If everything is clear, you can fill the prescription."

In my mind, I thought, *"Okay no problem. I'm not having any weird gynecological symptoms."* Hence, I scheduled an appointment with the front desk to have the ultrasound done the following Friday.

We've all been there when the technician does the testing; whether X-Rays, ultrasounds or what-have-you. We try to read their faces. I asked the kind girl dressed in blue medical scrubs, "Do you see anything? Does everything look okay?"

She did not have a good poker face. Of course, the medical staff are trained to give patients the same, generic, canned response. "Sorry, you're going to have to get the results from your doctor."

"Please, I can tell by the look on your face…" I pushed. She would not budge.

"I can't, Juliet. It's not my place. You'll have to talk to the doc."

However, I noticed her keen interest in what was on the screen. Out of curiosity, she asked, "Have you ever had any type of cyst before? Or any other gynecological problem?"

I shook my head. "No, nothing. My period has been like clockwork. I get it every 29 days and have ever since I was 13. No pain, no cysts. I've never even had very bad menstrual cycles." It was true. *'Down there*' everything had been A-Okay with me throughout my entire life. However, the expression on her face and that question she asked left me with a sense of doubt.

As I got dressed and ready to leave the appointment, I began to wonder. *'Was there something wrong? Had she spotted something bad on the ultrasound? Why had she asked me that question?'*

For about an hour after my appointment, I worried and fretted. I had anxiety, fears and many strange questions running through my mind. Just as easily as they had been planted, I quickly chased those thoughts right out of my head. Worry and anxiety was not going to serve me well! Besides, I considered myself to be in top physical health. I was a nonfat foodie and Diet Coke-drinking girl. I was a workout queen, running six days a week and hitting the gym four or more days. Externally, I was a picture of good health.

There was nothing that would stop me from enjoying the family trip I had planned with my daughter and our big family. We were leaving the very next day, a Saturday, on a trip to the Sierra Nevada Mountains. My parents, siblings and their families were also going camping for the next nine days. As any mother knows, taking a big journey with the family – especially a camping trip – requires a lot of extra packing and attention to detail. For goodness sake, you must plan everything from the best and lightest shoes to wear hiking, to the nitty gritty details of the graham crackers and marshmallows for the s'mores. There was no time to think about 'what-ifs' or hypothetical illnesses.

Our family rolled out as planned the next day. We had a fabulous time seeing the beautiful mountains, rafting down the Truckee River and plenty of one-on-one with Mother Nature. We survived the high altitude of the Sierra Mountains with no issues. No one got lost, injured or separated from the group. We saw a lot of wildlife and had a family vacation to remember. It was exactly what I needed at the time to clear my mind from the worry and anxiety that can take over one's psyche.

Upon returning the following week on a late Sunday night with my best friend Miles, there was a yellow note on my door from the post office. It was a notice of a certified letter from my OB-GYN's office that was pending pickup. When I saw the sender's address on that post office notification, I froze. At that moment, I knew with 100% certainty that something was seriously wrong.

"Miles, Miles! Oh my goodness, something's wrong. Doctors' offices don't send certified letters unless there's something major."

Ever the kind and caring friend, as well as being a doctor, Miles explained the protocol at most clinics. "Juliet, sometimes we just have to send letters out like that to let people know their results are all good. You shouldn't get so worked up over this, at least not yet."

Deep down, I knew that Miles was only trying to make me feel better. I had never received a certified letter from any doctor's office just to tell me that my results were all good.

To make matters worse, I was amid a messy divorce. I was supposed to appear in court for the divorce hearing at 8:45 a.m. on Monday morning. The doctor's office did not open until 9:00 a.m. Therefore, the timing of this medical issue could not have been more awkward.

As I tucked my five-year old daughter into bed that night, we prayed together. I carried the sudden feeling of burden, sadness, and uneasiness inside my mind, like a wall of bricks that stacks against your mental well-being.

My woes were twofold; I bore the emotional sadness of my marriage ending, as well as the anguish of not knowing my health issue. My thoughts gripped me with insatiable fear.

"Get off it, Juliet," I kept telling myself. *"Stop going on the crazy train, Juliet. You don't know anything until you talk to your doctor. Just get through the divorce. One dilemma at a time."*

I rose early to drop my daughter off at school at 8:15 a.m., then left for the courthouse to wait for the divorce hearing. I sat in court as my divorce was being finalized. I felt so sad, the love of my life and man that I had loved so much was gone. As a married couple, we did not work very well together. Upon leaving the courthouse, I remember getting in the car and crying over the finality of our marriage. All of our hopes and dreams were shattered.

Finally, I pulled myself together and drove out of the courthouse. On the way home, I remembered to call my OB-GYN, which I did while driving on the freeway *(which I don't recommend, by the way)*. The secretary put the doctor on the phone.

"Juliet, are you sitting down?" she asked.

"Yes," I replied. "I'm driving, so I'm definitely sitting down."

"Listen, your test came back. There was a cyst with a tumor inside. I can say with 90% certainty that it is cancer."

I was stunned. A shockwave coursed through my body. "What? What did you just say?" I had to find somewhere to pull over quickly.

"I said... that I think it's cancer," my doctor repeated. I started crying. "I'm so sorry, Juliet, but you need to do some things right away. You need to get a blood test and an MRI. I'm going to give you the names of the testing clinics. You need to please go to these labs and do it right now."

After we hung up, I drove immediately to my sister Jennifer's house, crying the entire way. I wondered how I would even get there, as I could barely see past the tears and eyeliner that had welled up in my eyes. When I arrived, my sister held me in her arms as I cried. Fear paralyzed my body and mind. However, I did exactly what my doctor asked and went the very same day to get the lab tests and MRI. Meanwhile, I had to wait for the test results.

CA 125 is a protein that is a supposed biomarker or tumor marker. CA 125 can be found in greater concentration in ovarian cancer cells than in other cells, therefore it enables doctors to know whether you have cancer or not. My CA 125 markers came back high.

My doctor then referred me to an oncologist, whereupon I met with Dr. Bahador. He was known as one of the best OB-GYN oncologists in the world (*literally*). Dr. Bahador had incredible bedside manner and was so nice and kind as he explained things to me. He told me that I needed to have surgery and then afterwards, he would know what stage I was at and if the cancer had spread to other parts of my body. My family and friends rallied around me. Miles, Mary, Parvaneh, Joan and Heidi offered friendship and support.

A week later, I was about to check into the hospital for the surgery. On the night before, I decided to clear my head with a vigorous run. I remember lying down on the grass and looking up at the stars. This was my one-on-one with God. "God, are you there? I need to know... I need to know if I'm going to live through this. God, *please!* I'm a single mother with a five-year-old. Help me!" I begged God to hear me, but the twilight eve was silent.

After a good cry, I suddenly felt a surge of peace wash over me. Then, I heard God speak to me in my heart. Very quietly and softly, he said, "Trust in me that I will take care of you, Juliet."

In that moment, I knew that I would be okay. No matter what hardships came at me, I knew that I would live. So, the very next morning, I went nervously – yet knowingly – into robotic surgery. During the last few seconds before the anesthesiologist carefully counted down the seconds, my last few, fleeting thoughts were of wonder and fear of the unknown.

"Will I wake up and hear the doctor say the cancer is not that bad, or will he tell me it is Stage 5?" I wondered. *"Juliet, you only have a few weeks to live..."*

My thoughts jumped back and forth from one side of my brain to the other, like a seesaw at a children's playground. Then, I remembered God. *"Trust what you heard from God, Juliet."* That inner voice outweighed the fear and panic.

As any mother would probably feel if she were in the same situation – which perhaps you are – the most rampant and continuous thoughts were of my dear little girl. I hoped that my child would not have to witness her mother's death. I could not help but to wonder what that would do to her – at the tender and vulnerable age of five – if she were to lose me? I was her main source of stability and comfort.

Just as the anesthesia kicked in, I yelled to God in my thoughts. "Okay God! I put my life, my child and my everything into your hands. I surrender to you." Then, my eyes grew heavy and dark, as I fell into the deep tunnels of my subconscious.

A few hours later, I blinked under the bright lights of the fluorescent ceiling. It was bright and I felt woozy and groggy.

"Good afternoon! Juliet, can you hear me?"

I nodded. It was Dr. Bahador. He had returned to check on my recovery.

"I just wanted to give you an update," he stated. "First, everything went well. You are okay. Your tumor was very small, but we had a difficult time testing the tumor in surgery."

"So, what does that mean?" I asked.

"Well, I'm going to have to send it off to Stanford University for a clear diagnosis. It may take several weeks before we get the most accurate results," he replied.

Obviously, I took that as a good sign, because at least the cancer had not spread to other places in my body. However, waiting six weeks for the prognosis was more than agonizing. *(Can you imagine?)*

THEN, THE CALL!! Dr. Bahador hit me with a literal 'wake-up call', *slap-you-in -the- face* reality check. "I received your results back from Stanford. You have ovarian cancer clear cell carcinoma. It's the most aggressive form of ovarian cancer you can have. In all the years I've been an oncologist, I've only seen one clear cell carcinoma in Stage 1C."

Yet, Dr. Bahador went on. "As you know, the cyst broke during surgery and there were cancer cells in the washing of your abdomen. Because of that, you will require three rounds of chemotherapy. And because it's the worst, most aggressive kind of cancer, you're going to need a double dose of chemotherapy each time."

Typically, cancer treatments only require one dose of chemotherapy per session. However, for this type of cancer, the doctors went after it just as tenaciously as the cancer cells themselves. I imagined us attacking those cells! Die cancer, die!

Later, Dr. Bahador disclosed that if I had come to see him even 12 weeks later, it would have been too late in the game to make an impact. Although not impossible, it would have been much tougher to beat if the cancer had progressed to Stage 5. It was officially diagnosed as ovarian cancer clear cell carcinoma Stage 1C. For me, the comparable survival rate was approximately 87% within five years.

What does that mean? According to the American Cancer Society's standards, that means surviving for at least five years after the treatment is over and my body goes into remission. Apparently, if you survive for five years after cancer, you're pretty much '*in the clear*'.

Out of 100 women that are diagnosed with ovarian cancer clear cell carcinoma at this stage, 87 women will live up to 5 years and 13 of them will die within those 5 years.

Next, I embarked upon the difficulties of setting up my life around chemotherapy. I no longer had a husband to help me, so I had to figure out who would take care of my daughter and who would take care of me. Part of me was too scared to start chemo; perhaps even more than when I had surgery. I knew there were a lot of people that died because of chemotherapy. However, I also knew there were many more that lived.

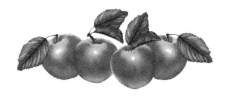

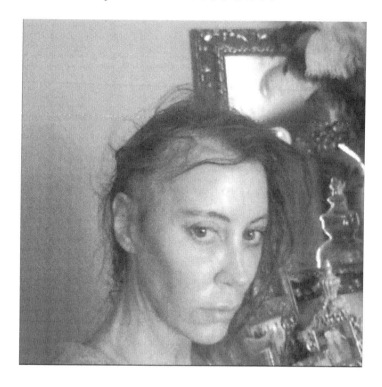

After feeling the sharp prick in my skin from the IV needle, the chemicals traveled through my vein and shot through my entire body. I knew there was no turning back. I wanted everything that modern medicine could give me to get well and healthy again, but I also developed an insatiable appetite for knowledge. Like a sponge, I absorbed as much information I could learn about cancer. I read books, articles, medical journals and any literature I could find. I studied the moves of other cancer survivors to learn what they did or didn't do.

However, it was rather difficult to find good, clear information that was easy to digest. This was indeed one of the most emotionally stressful times in my life. How could I begin to wrap myself around trying to process and learn the overwhelming amount of material? It was just plain hard,but I knew my life depended upon it.

First I wondered, "Have I done anything, in any way, to contribute to this cancer?" Although my doctor and others warned me not to blame myself, I needed to find out what part in this I could have avoided or done differently, just as anyone might wonder. This was a pivotal point between questioning *'Why did this happen to me?'* and *'What did I ever do to deserve this?'*

Just to be straight, no one deserves cancer! However, these inquisitions helped me to cope and look at the cancer from a different perspective. Like wearing a new pair of glasses, I was now going to view this cancer thing from a totally different angle. From destitute to survival, I told myself I would become a survivor. Remembering that calm, clear, peaceful voice from God as I lay on the green grass the night before my surgery... I repeated what he said. "Juliet, you will not die."

Now it was my time to do my part. I said aloud, "Modern medicine you do your part and I will figure out my part." So, I literally immersed myself into the "C" word to discover, read and dissect the material for maximum comprehension.

Ladies and Gents, there is a revelation I must disclose to you. Suzanne Somers refers to it as the 'Tipping Point'. She went from breast cancer survivor to cancer activist and health advocate. The best way I can explain the tipping point is when the body's normal cells start to mutate into cancer cells. However, I like to call it the imperfect storm.

You see, we all have cancer cells in our body, everyday. Shocking, right?! It just comes down to any day or moment in time that those cancer cells start to mutate. If they've been exposed to enough toxins, chemicals and not enough nutrition, my belief is that the cells mutate. Furthermore, if the body continuously gets fed bad stuff, those cancer cells begin to grow.

Before my cancer diagnosis, I'll admit that I was all about the 99 cent grocery bargains. Oh yes, I threw tons of processed foods in my cart. Of course, I'd throw a few pieces of pesticide-filled fruit in there too, but rarely any vegetables. I was a single mother trying to make a house payment and support my daughter and myself. If food was cheap and fast, I bought it. Of course, it also had to be low calorie and non-fat, because I was all about the 'skinny' look. My clueless self never minded that all these diet foods were filled with loads of chemicals and artificial sweeteners. All I cared about was that I was going to be skinny.

As I learned and studied, I realized that I was feeding my body tons of processed foods filled with all GMOs, chemicals and tons of hidden sugars. On top of it, I was eating artificial sweeteners like they were going out of style. Little did I know, these are CARCINOGENIC. I must have drank five Diet Cokes a day, not to mention all the Sweet n' Lows that I used in my water and cereal. I was also a nonfat, artificial yogurt freak. I literally went to those yogurt shops twice a day to eat chocolate, frozen yogurt that was filled with artificial flavors, sweeteners and dyes. Admittedly, my diet had no nutritional value at all. My poor, poor body!

To make matters worse, the marriage I had just ended was extremely toxic and caused me a lot of emotional stress. This carried its own set of negative chemicals in the body. But that wasn't all! A lot of prescription drugs that I had been taking were also toxic, along with as many as five Tylenol P.M.'s that I took to help me sleep at night because of the turmoil from the ending of my marriage and the stress of being a single mother. When I discovered how damaging these were to my liver, I was stunned.

As Charlotte Gerson from the Gerson Therapy says, "With a toxic body, you get sick. But with a toxic liver, you get cancer." Gerson Therapy is the largest holistic approach to healing and curing cancer in the world.

As I continued reading and digesting all this information, I began to realize that most of the beauty, hair care products and perfumes we consume are also filled with hazardous and toxic chemicals. The beauty industry exceeds over 600 billion dollars a year, and yet it has very few FDA restrictions on what ingredients can or cannot be used. Yet, it was so easy to be beautiful with chemicals, that's for damn sure!

During my cancer treatment and research, it came to my attention that there were several other people on my street that had cancer at the same time as me. In fact, within a thirty-house neighborhood, at least fifteen people had cancer at the same time. Within a six-house radius of mine, five women (including myself) all had cancer! The neighbor to my left and the lady to my right both had cancer. I knew there had to be a connecting link, it was simply too coincidental.

"I need to put on my 'Erin Brockovich' hat and get to work here," I told one of the neighbors. I searched the area where we lived, yet couldn't find any solid evidence of a toxic source. Then, it suddenly hit me. We lived on a golf course. In fact, the street that we lived on had a golf course on either side.

"Don't they spray a lot of fertilizers to keep the greens so beautiful?" I wondered. Instantly, I jumped on the quest for answers. I called the golf course and they told me that they spray fungicides, mildewcides, pesticides, herbicides and a ton of other stuff. Not to mention, twice a year, they killed off the grass by using tons of chemicals. Then, they reseeded it with an

additional load of hazardous sprays during the fall and spring months.

Feeling disgusted by this news, I asked, "How many times a week do you spray?"

"Oh, three or four times early in the morning before most people are awake," he knowingly replied.

"Well, you have a city-owned golf course. Can you give me a list of all the stuff you spray? Can I talk to the superintendent of the golf course?" I asked.

"He's out on a leave of absence right now."

"Oh, really?" I stated. "Is he okay?"

"No," he replied quietly. "I'm afraid he has cancer."

I was floored. "Don't you think it's a little strange how a lot of the people in this community have cancer? With so many pesticides and toxic chemicals being sprayed every day?"

"Well, ma'am, all the stuff that we spray is all approved by the FDA to spray on fruits and vegetables and crops."

'FDA my ass', I thought to myself.

"Well, the bottom line is that nobody lives right in the middle of a crop, do they?" I retorted. Although it was not this guy's fault exclusively, I was angry that this stuff was allegedly legal and that no one was doing anything about it. This news was enough for me to put my house up for sale. I did not need to be subjected to any more chemicals while I was recovering and trying to stay cancer-free.

Although I tried to share the knowledge with my neighbors, no one seemed to have any interest or belief in what I had to say. You must be your own advocate. Unfortunately, we can't blame the doctors, as they are not trained in a lot of nutrition or prevention tactics, if any at all.

On a lighter note – I have discovered a common denominator between all my research – and that is what I am about to tell you. Organic living and eating a plant-based diet is the absolute best method of cancer prevention. Your mama was right! She wasn't kidding... you *should* be eating your vegetables!

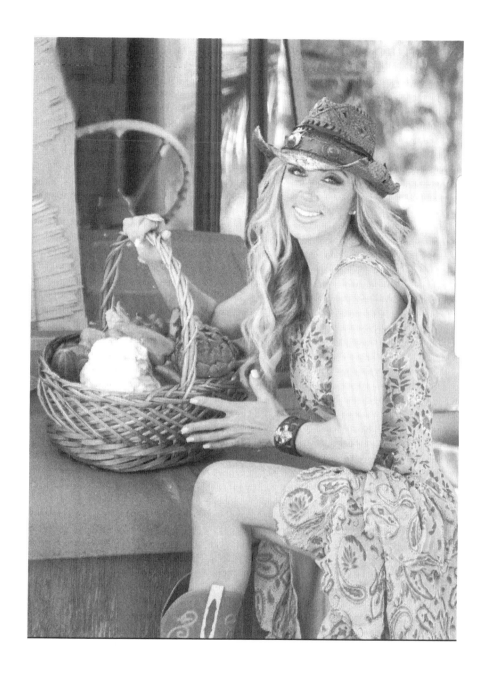

Chapter Two

What I Do

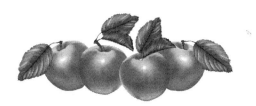

Ready, steady, go! Alrighty, this is what I do do do do do. *Isn't that a Katy Perry song?*

Before I delve into the crux of the next phase, I just want to warn you that this is *not really* Chapter Two. At least, not in the sense that you're expecting. My goal in providing you with this information – this knowledge, if you will – is not just to talk about the cancer ordeal that I went through. God forbid you may be going through this too, however, if you may have recently found out you have cancer, then please listen to me very closely and "DO" just like I do.

Just a little thought as we move forward: Strive to live and eat healthier. I'm not perfect here, so I'm not going to proclaim that if you eat something bad, you may get cancer. That's simply not the case. Or just because you were exposed to some kind of toxin when you were twelve does not mean you will get cancer, either. What we want to strive for is a healthier body and life. Progress, not perfection.

I also want to share that there are other factors that play a role in the risk of one's individual predisposition to cancer. There's a genetic component, environmental, and what I believe is also just called "Our Time" when God decides to take us home. Again, this is just my personal belief, and you are entitled to any/all of your own views regarding this topic.

Hence, you can do a lot of things to lower your risk of getting cancer, surviving cancer or having a reoccurrence. However, sometimes, there are factors that you may not even be privy to. For example, someone who buys or leases a home that was filled with asbestos. Or in my case, living directly on a golf course that constantly and unknowingly sprayed tons of pesticides, fungicides and herbicides.

There may be people living in a home, right now, that is filled with dangerous molds, bacteria or other cancer-causing toxins. The families may have installed new flooring that was sprayed with formaldehyde, and many other external hazards. There are hundreds of stories like these.

Right now, there may be people working at a factory that sprays certain types of chemicals that cause cancer and/or other industries that have harmful toxic chemicals. It's not just our homes we need to worry about, but the places we work and the activities we do every day. Cancer doesn't selectively choose people. I believe it is a culmination of all the environmental and physical hazards that we unknowingly face, each and every day of life.

When you start to educate yourself and really see what you're putting on your body and hair, or the fumes you breathe in whenever you clean your home, it is shocking! Like a revelation, you will become enlightened and awakened. You'll likely stop short in your tracks and say, "*Wow! I can't believe that I exposed myself to so many toxic things, situations, personal care products, foods and even people...*"

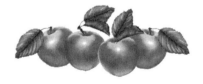

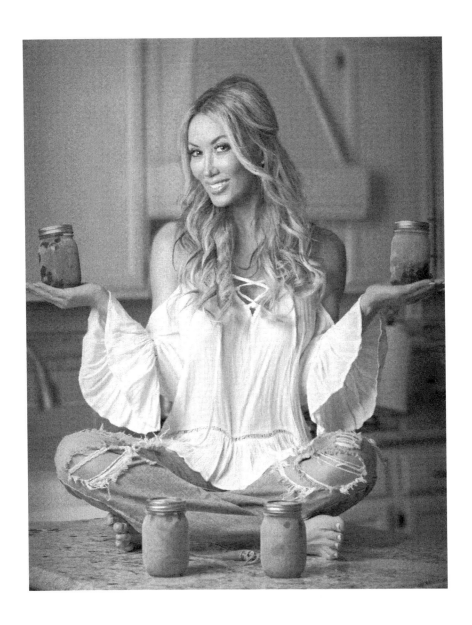

Here's the story of my daily routine. This is what I do every day, as a cancer survivor, with the hope of decreasing my odds of reoccurrence.

1. I strive to get eight hours of sleep each night, but sometimes it ends up being seven. For me, sleep is extremely important. I do whatever it takes to get a sound sleep, including wearing a dark sleep mask and having dark drapes in my room. I also sleep with an air purifier. Rabbit Air is my preference. Your bedroom is one of the places that you spend the most time, therefore while you sleep you should make sure that the air you're breathing is free of any pollution or toxins. Rabbit Air purifiers work well, yet without the huge price tag. For those who cannot afford hospital-grade homes that purify all the air, this is the best way to go. There was a study at Harvard that noted the air found in homes is more polluted than the toxins found in the air outside. WHAT? Yes, that's right... so all those chemicals we use to clean our homes can be

extremely toxic, as well as perfumes, hairspray, aerosol air fresheners, and the list goes on.

2. As soon as I rise, I thank God that I'm alive and for this day. Then, I read a small passage from one of my inspirational books to get my mind going in the right direction.

3. Next, I let the light into my darkened room. Drawing back my curtains, I let the sun shine in and then go around the rest of the house to do the same. I also open the windows to let in the fresh air. Why do I do this? Getting Vitamin D is very important. There's a link between low Vitamin D levels and cancer, so flip those shades on your eyes and let some sun shine on your face. Humans get a lot of Vitamin D through our eyes.

4. I make my bed first thing in the morning. This is part of good sleep habits. Bad sleep habits include not making the bed, using the phone in bed, etc. Don't get under the covers until you're ready to go to sleep because you are sending signals to the brain when you have a routine for when you go to sleep and when to wake up. Hence, making the bed and

opening the drapes sends the signals to my brain that sleep time is over and it's time to start the day! There have been a lot of studies linking good sleep routines and how it helps people sleep better, so those who have trouble sleeping should try this.

5. Next, I get into my workout wear and do about 5 – 10 minute meditation. It's hard for me to get into that quiet place, but I highly recommend it. I use positive affirmations or music.

6. Once the meditation session is over, I start my yoga routine and scan my body to try to determine which areas feel tight and where the energy is. Ask your body, "Where do you hurt?" and it will tell you, so go to that area and stretch and massage it. Love it!

7. Once the mini-yoga session is over, I'm ready to fill my body with something good. I start out with 16 oz. of lukewarm lemon water. The water I drink is Palomar Mountain Spring Water. You should try to find the purest water in your area and have it delivered to your house for maximum convenience. The lemon cleanses the body and the liver of any

extra toxic waste that has been released while you slept; it can be flushed out.

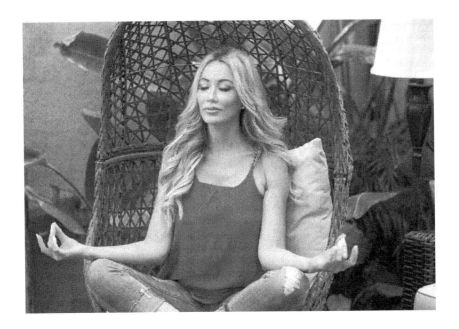

8. Each morning, I walk over to my medicine cabinet. I try to make things super easy because the easier it is, the more likely it will get done. I take one multivitamin with 3000 milligrams of Vitamin C, Vitamin Q10 and Vitamin D. Once each week, I also take an iron pill. Sublingual Vitamin B12. You cannot take it orally because the body does not absorb it. So, I get it in a shot or take it underneath my tongue. That's the only way the body can absorb it.

9. For food, I start with three fresh juices, using one carrot and two Gerson Therapy green juices. I drink them half an hour apart.

10. After drinking one fresh carrot juice and one green juice, I cook my gluten-free, organic oatmeal. It just wouldn't be the same without a dash of walnuts, as these are considered an 'almighty' brain nut with a lot of healthy omegas. Add a dash of cinnamon, because it regulates your blood sugar all day long. You could opt for a sprinkle of blueberries and a tablespoon of chia seeds and/or hemp seeds. Personally, I prefer a little bit of organic Stevia sweetener and/or coconut milk, too. I should add that everything I use is organic!

11. Now for the hard part. You can do it anyway you like, but as tough as it is, you've got to get that dose of apple cider vinegar. I just go for a fast, quick and easy swig of organic apple cider vinegar mixed with some turmeric and black pepper. When you read the '*Do's and Don'ts*' section, you'll understand why. I take it from the powdered form, but I know lots of people that do take turmeric pills.

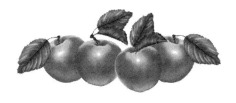

When the body is toxic, people get disease and sicknesses. When the liver is toxic, people get cancer.

~ Charlotte Gerson

NOTE: Please read Gerson Therapy Handbook first before doing coffee enema. Also, consult your doctor first.

12. Deep breath for this one. It's tough to talk about. The preparation of my coffee enema (*which actually takes place the night before*) is not something I like to talk to everyone about, but nevertheless, it is a very important part of my day that I cannot righteously leave out.

So, folks, here it is: I take 1 quart of distilled water and 3 large tablespoons of ground, organic coffee. Boil them for 3 minutes and then turn on low heat to simmer for 15 minutes. I find it easier to prepare this the night before, so that when I wake up and drink my juices, it is working as a detox for my body. The coffee has obviously cooled down by morning and is ready for me to use. So, people... most of you drink your coffee. Brace yourself for the way I drink coffee, as it may be difficult to imagine. It's a coffee enema! There, I said it. What a relief. I'll bet you've never had Starbucks coffee like this before. 😊 Before you say, "*What the...?*" let me explain why.

While you are juicing and detoxing the cells, all the dead cells and toxins that were in the cells get flushed into the bloodstream. The liver is the filtering system of our bodies. Every three minutes, the entire network of blood that flows through our bodies from our brains to our little toes cycles through the liver. Therefore, if your liver is not functioning at 100%, then it will not be able to rid the blood from all the toxins.

Charlotte Gerson, who was the daughter of Max Gerson (*founder of the Gerson Therapy*), says that when the body is toxic, people get diseases and other illnesses. But with a toxic liver, people get cancer.

Throughout her 96 years of life, Charlotte continued her father's work by opening up Gerson clinics around the globe; to treat patients holistically. The Gerson Therapy is the largest known holistic approach to healing cancer in the world. At the time of publishing this book, Charlotte is alive and well, retired and living in San Diego, California. To me, this long lifespan has a lot to do with the healthy lifestyle she leads, and certainly she has set an example to both cancer and non-cancer survivors.

At any rate, you want to make sure that you're keeping your liver at its optimal working capacity. The coffee enema helps to support the liver. The purpose of the enema is to remove toxins which have accumulated in the liver; and to remove free radicals from the bloodstream. Researchers found that the caffeine travels via the hemorrhoidial vein and the portal system to the liver opens the bile ducts, allowing the liver to release bile that contains toxins. It then dumps the toxins back into the colon, where it can continue with its eventual elimination. I guess you could call it the "process of elimination" in a literal sense.

To learn how to do a coffee enema, go to my website: puregirlinatoxicworld.com. There's lots of benefits, which you will find in my do's and don'ts section. And if you think this is some new deal, think again! This method dates to around 1600 B.C. I personally think it's best to do this after a bowel movement when your colon track is fairly clean. If you have not had a good, old-fashioned poop, then you can first clean yourself out with a little distilled water in the enema bag and then eliminate.

Just before you begin, you need to drink 16 oz. of organic coconut water or Vitamin Water Zero Revive. The reason for this is because the coffee enema disturbs the electrolyte balance in your system, and the electrolytes in the water replenishes them. I do this for about 12 – 15 minutes and then it's all done. I can't tell you how great I feel after doing this.

13. I reward myself by eating a green apple, although I don't eat too much fruit, since it tends to have a lot of sugar. Sugar feeds cancer and candida. So, I normally eat only a couple of pieces of fruit each day.

14. Sometimes for lunch I'll have a big blend of vegetables in my Blend Tec blender with some pea protein or, I'll eat some tofu and a salad. Sunflower

CANCER? WE'VE GOT THIS!

seed butter on quinoa crackers is another good lunch. When you become a vegan, there's a ton of recipe books and ideas you can find online.

15. Either with lunch or sometime in the afternoon, I drink three cups of green tea caffeine-free, with Pau d'Arco tea. It is an invaluable anti-cancer tea. I prepare this in the morning with my oatmeal and put it in a large, stainless-steel 24 oz. container. Simply boil water with some lemon juice and a little Stevia sweetener. You can even sip it throughout the day, whenever you want to feel hydrated.

16. Just like the rest of the households across America, dinner is very important to me. I eat a huge salad with all sorts of colored vegetables or a yummy, hot vegetable dish. One of my favorites is the vegan eggplant parmesan, or I might enjoy some veggies cooked in coconut curry ginger sauce. Variety is the key here – so choose a rainbow of vegetables at the farmer's market or some other type of organic vegetable stand – and then find some great recipes to make new, exciting dishes. In fact, you can find many suggested vegan cookbooks on my website.

17. Did I mention that at night I eat a humungous salad that could probably feed a family of four? On that note, I typically make my own dressing. It consists of two tablespoons of flaxseed oil, some veganaise, garlic, some other spices and a dash of lemon juice.

18. Just before I go to bed, I take 3,000mg of Vitamin C and another 50mcg of Vitamin D with a tablespoon of apple cider vinegar mixed with turmeric and black pepper. I do this about two hours before going to bed.

19. Literally, just before I turn off the lights, I take a couple of probiotic tablets. This is one of the most important things you can do, but you must take the probiotic on an empty stomach and at night because it can build your gut flora while you sleep. If not, you will just be flushing them out during the day with food and water. At the same time, I take two supplements of turkey tail mushroom and Cell Forte Max 3. You'll discover more about these in the do's and don'ts.

20. When I lie down, one of the last things I do is take 6mg of melatonin and Relaxall. They offer some

good, natural herbs that help to quiet the brain down at night.

Because of the ovarian cancer, I had to undergo a hysterectomy. Since that surgery, I noticed that I have been unable to sleep as well as I did prior to having my 'woman parts' removed. I'm not sure if there is any correlation, but I have read and researched a lot of different studies about sleep.

As I mentioned earlier, one of the most effective ways they have found in obtaining a good, quality night's sleep is in the sleep behavior and routines. Basically, this is another term for training your brain to go to sleep by sending it certain signals. You must also do the same behaviors when you get up in the morning, as your internal psyche will tell the body that it's time to wake up now! Therefore, one of the most important things you should do is make a routine for each night before you go to bed. In contrast, one of the worst things you can do is lie in bed under your covers and watch TV or be on the phone or your computer. It is okay to have the bed fully made and lie on top of the blankets, so long as you are not in "just about to go to sleep mode".

I'm not big on taking any prescription pills because they're toxic to the body. However, sometimes if I'm really in need of a sleep aid, I have two diphenhydramine HCl 25 mg on hand. Please just take the sleep aid itself, and never Tylenol PM. This is very damaging to the liver and extremely toxic. Remember toxic bodies make us sick, but toxic livers bring on cancer.

However, I want to stress to you the importance of doing most of these things in sequence. Try not to skip them. That is why I have numbered them for you.

Remember, sleep is critical to the body and mind for healing. That is when it goes into healing damaged cells and building our immune systems, etc. Finally, I turn off the light and climb underneath the blankets. Ahhh... I love that moment.

Chapter Three

If You Are Currently Going Through Chemo & Radiation

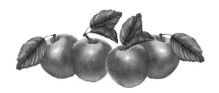

If you have cancer and are currently in chemotherapy or radiation treatment, there are some things you should not do. When you read Chapter Four and Five, some of the following points will not apply to you, however, after you are finished with chemo and radiation, I will recommend that you re-read these chapters and add them to your list of do's and don'ts. Certain things require a strong immune system and during the chemotherapy, your body will be at its most vulnerable state because undergoing chemotherapy puts you at a very high risk for infection. Your body simply may not be able to fight it off at this time.

On that note, I want to mention that I'm a huge supporter of the Gerson Therapy. I suggest that you also look into this. If you decide to do the Gerson Therapy, you must stick with it for two to three years after your cancer is gone, if not longer. Some of the do's and don'ts you will read about in the next two chapters are not suggestions by the Gerson Therapy.

Personally speaking, I did the Gerson Therapy *after* I had chemotherapy. I did it for two years, and now I do what is referred to as an 80/20 lifestyle. That means you eat and live 80% Gerson Therapy and the remaining 20% what you want.

Also, I must share with you that I am *not a doctor,* nor a nutritionist. I'm just a cancer survivor who is sharing my journey and what I've studied over the last five years. The bottom line is this: I could get cancer again and you could get cancer again, even after doing all of these things. Despite both of us doing all the do's and don'ts exactly, there are other factors in life we cannot control.

For example, both you and I could be exposed to a toxin in our environment that we are unaware of that causes cancer. This happens all the time and it is very sad, but it is something we do not have control over. Secondly, there is a genetic factor. Yes, it may only be 10%, but if you have a genetic mutation, there's not too much you could do about your DNA. It is without question that these two things alone can greatly increase your odds of getting cancer or of reoccurrence.

Finally, there is what I like to call the "God Factor". If it's your time, it's your time. My belief is that God is the giver of life and God is the taker of life. If we want to live, we must do whatever we can to survive, and I do know for a fact that doing these do's and don'ts will greatly decrease your odds of getting cancer and/or of having it come back even if you do get it. Committing to do these do's and don'ts will also help you beat the odds of dying from cancer, so you have nothing to lose by applying them to your everyday routine.

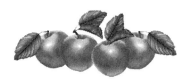

Don'ts for Those Currently Going Through Chemo & Radiation:

1. **DON'T:** Do not eat raw fruits and veggies. Fruits are okay if they are first washed with a non-toxic soap, such as Dr. Bronzer's Baby Soap. They should be peeled. If you can't peel it, you can't eat it. Vegetables should also be washed and cooked. You can eat loads of veggies that are steamed, sauteed, or baked any way you like, as long as they're cooked.

Why? Fresh fruits and vegetables can have germs and bacteria on the outside, which can cause illness. When a person is going through cancer treatment, their immune system is extremely compromised. It may not have the ability to fight off an infection.

2. **DON'T:** Don't share bath towels or drinking glasses with anyone.

Why? People have bacteria and viruses that can get into your body while your system is weak.

3. **DON'T:** Don't travel. Also, avoid large crowds of people, such as schools, malls, and public gatherings. If you must go, wear masks.

Why? You could come into contact with more germs, viruses, and bacterias.

4. **DON'T:** Don't be around any crops, golf courses, or flower fields.

Why? These environments are often sprayed with heavy chemicals, pesticides, and fertilizers; which can compromise your immune system even more.

5. DON'T: Do not clean up droppings from your pet, birdcage, litter box, fish tanks, or dog wee-wee pads. Don't even change any baby diapers.

Why? The bacteria from these items could cause an infection.

6. DON'T: Do not play, walk, or swim in ponds, lakes, rivers, or water parks.

Why? The water found in these places carries a high amount of viruses and bacterias. They can be deadly to you at this point.

7. DON'T: Don't use razor blades.

Why? Use an electric razor instead. It's not worth cutting yourself and exposing your skin to an open wound.

8. DON'T: Ladies, during this time of cancer treatment, do not use tampons, vaginal suppositories, or douches.

Why? You run the risk of getting an infection.

Chapter Four

Do's

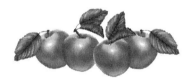

Whenever I meet people and get the opportunity to converse face-to-face, I am happy to share my journey and experience. In fact, I want to tell as many people as possible. By helping others who may be going through this – or who have loved ones that are suffering – I feel as though I may be comforting them. Overcoming this terrible, awful disease has become my newfound passion. Cancer? We Got This!

Like you, I was clueless about all of the 'things' lurking out there, things we all use everyday as common household products. Many of them are toxic, yet the general public remains unaware and largely ignorant of the grim reality. TV ads and expensive marketing campaigns help to sell these products. The only way to avoid them and to decrease your odds of getting cancer is to empower yourself with knowledge.

That is what this little book is all about. I want you to have the knowledge and the power to defeat cancer. I have already researched and applied this awareness to my own life, and thankfully, it worked. Whenever people ask me questions regarding personal care products, foods, or lifestyle, they are sometimes shocked to discover a favorite item or brand they have been using for a long time is not good for them.

Just to be clear, I am not dissing any companies, corporations, or individuals. All of these do's and don'ts are backed by thorough research and studies completed by scientists, doctors and cancer researchers. The more we know about cancer, the greater our chances will be for survival.

Please take my book with you on your next shopping expedition. Show it to your friends and family. Let's say goodbye and good riddance to cancer.

Before we get into the specific do's and don'ts, I want to give you the definition of CARCINOGENIC. I will talk about CARCINOGENICS a lot, so you must know what it means. Simply put, CARCINOGENICS are substances that can lead to cancer.

Now, without further "A DO" ...

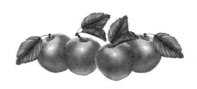

1. DO: Opt for natural sugars, such as fruit juices, stevia, guava nectar, honey, molasses, and maple sugar. Choose all organic.

Why?   Refined sugar feeds cancer cells; even natural sugars. Therefore, you want to keep sugar intake on the low scale.

2. DO: Try to stop and breathe, literally!

Why?   Deep breathing a couple of times each day brings oxygen to the cells, and cancer does not like oxygen. Deliberate breathing will help calm you down and bring nutrients to your organs.

3. DO: Get some Vitamin D – either from the sun – or by taking Vitamin D supplements. Do this every day.

Why?   There is a link between low vitamin D levels and cancer.

4. DO: Drink mountain spring water. I use Palomar Mountain Spring water. It comes in BPA-free bottles. You could also use a professional grade filtering system, but the filter should be changed every 3–6 months.

Why?   Spring water does not have any chemicals in it.

5. DO: Get a whole water filter for your entire house – if you can afford it – or at least get a shower water filter. These are available at Home Depot for about $30. These also need to changed every 3–6 months.

Why?   This may come as a surprise, but water in most neighborhoods has chemicals, chlorine and even prescription drugs (*believe it or not*)! It only takes 29 seconds for something you put on your skin to get into your bloodstream.

6. DO: Drink from glass, ceramic, or stainless steel water bottles.

Why?   Plastic water bottles have BPA, which is a chemical in plastic known to cause cancer. The chemicals get more absorbed into the water as it is frozen or heated up.

7. DO: If you do buy canned foods, make sure they are labeled "BPA Free", such as beans, etc. If it does not say that on the outside of the can, it is most likely lined with a toxic plastic that will seep into your food.

Why?   Refer to #6.

8. **DO:**   Cook with glass, porcelain, iron, or stainless steel.

Why?   Non-stick cookware is made with a chemical known as P.F.O.A., which emits toxic fumes that you inhale every time you cook. It also gets into your food. PFOA is linked to cancer.

9. **DO:**   Gerson Therapy. Get the Gerson Therapy handbook and study it.

Why?   It's the largest known holistic approach to healing cancer in the world. (If you have cancer and are undergoing chemotherapy at this time, you will need to cook your vegetables; no juicing. Your white cell count is low during chemotherapy and there are bacterias on raw fruits and vegetables. If you get sick, your body might not be strong enough to fight off a bacterial infection. You will have to wait to juice until you're done with chemo.)

10. **DO**   Go Vegan.

Why?   Numerous studies reveal that cancer rates among people who choose a plant-based diet are extremely low. Some studies say that *'going vegan'* after cancer cuts your risk of re-occurrence by 50% or greater.

11. **DO:** Eat only organic.

Why? If it's not organic, your food and beverages have chemicals, pesticides, herbicides, and other CARCINOGENIC toxins. At least 40 known CARCINOGENICS can be found in pesticides. Remember, you need to eliminate CARCINOGENICS.

12. **DO:** Keep a toxic-free home! Go to puregirlinatoxicworld.com to find toxic-free products and cleaning supplies for your household. Many things from laundry detergent to cleaners, personal care products, and other common items are toxic.

Why? Studies show that the air quality in our homes is actually more toxic than the air quality outside. Cleaning products have toxic chemicals in them. Some of them are extremely high on the cancer-causing scale, with loads of CARCINOGENICS. Let's chuck them in the trash can.

13. **DO:** Eat raw foods (After chemotherapy). These include living foods, greens, sprouts, vegetables, fruits, nuts, and seeds.

Why?   Raw foods are filled with chlorophyll, enzymes, vitamins, minerals, antioxidants, fiber, and phytonutrients. They also alkalize the entire system of the body. Disease cannot live in a Ph-balanced alkaline body.

14. **DO:**   Buy non-toxic, organic beauty products. This includes shampoos, conditioners, soaps, fluoride-free toothpastes, deodorants, shaving products, makeup, hair dyes, and skin care products.

Why?   The personal care products business is a billion-dollar industry with very few regulations. In fact, the word '*pure*', '*natural*' and '*non-toxic*' have no legal meaning when it comes to packaging. Yet, there are so many toxic chemicals in common personal care products. Some include lead, parabens, metals, formaldehyde, colors, dyes, and a huge list of CARCINOGENIC chemicals. Remember, CARCINOGENIC is boxed.

15. **DO:**   Wear toxic-free zinc sunscreen, hats, red or blue fabrics while you are out in the Sun. To find a list of healthy sunscreen choices, visit puregirlinatoxicworld.com.

Why?   Red and blue fabric gives significantly better protection from harmful UV rays. Melanoma can appear anywhere on the body, but more frequently in areas that are exposed to the sun, such as on hands, face, and neck.

16. **DO:** Eat Brazil nuts and walnuts.

Why? The Brazil-nut is packed with an anti-cancer property called selenium and powerful antioxidants. Walnuts have Omega 3's, fatty acids, and tons of antoxidants.

17. **DO:** Use the spice turmeric.

Why? Turmeric is one of the strongest weapons against cancer. Over 2,000 published studies have shown turmeric to actually stop cancer cells from dividing. Combining this with black pepper makes it even stronger. There are anti-inflammatory properties, along with many antioxidants.

18. **DO:** Use oregano.

Why? There are high levels of anti-oxidants and antimicrobial compounds. Oregano contains the photochemical quercetin, which may slow cancer growth.

19. **DO:** Lots of fresh ginger.

Why?   There are so many great health benefits in ginger, but just to name a few, it is an anti-inflammatory with a high amount of antoxidants. In laboratory studies, ginger extract has been shown to inhibit the growth of breast cancer cells. Another study confirmed that ginger can help in prevention of some cancers.

20. DO: Drink Pau d'Arco Tea.

Why?   Specifically, its use as a tool in the Gerson Therapy against cancer is powered by an active ingredient that produces a strong, biological response against cancer.

21. DO: Take nutritional yeast.

Why?   It's a complete amino acid that can be used as a good source of vegan protein. It is loaded with B vitamins, including B12. It has a plethora of minerals and vitamins, zinc, folic acid, fiber, and it even helps in detoxing the liver.

22. DO: Take organic, unfiltered apple cider vinegar, every day.

Why?   In some published studies, test tubes have revealed that vinegar can slow down the growth of cancer cells. It kills many types of bacteria, fungus, and lowers blood sugar levels. It also fights diabetes and can kill off candida.

23. **DO:** Take garlic every day in the amount of at least one clove.

Why? People who consume garlic on a daily basis had 30% fewer cancers. It also protects against some cancers, while reducing inflammation, boosting the immune system and naturally detoxifying the body.

24. **DO:** Turkey tail mushrooms, which you can get as a supplement.

Why? It has been shown to prevent cancer formation and growth of cancer cells. It also boosts the immune system.

25. **DO:** Organic, cold pressed flaxseed oil each day.

Why? It's packed with the Omega 3's, fatty acids, and lots of antoxidants. In some studies, flaxseed oil has shown to slow down the growth of cancerous tumors.

26. **DO:** Fresh Wheat grass shots. 1–2 oz. a day. If it makes you feel nauseous, that is good because it means that it's detoxing your

body. That should be a clue that your body is toxic and you need to get on a program of cleansing and detoxing.

Why?   It has cancer protection properties and is a detoxifier. It cleans out the liver and kidneys, while purifying the blood. It also has strong anti-inflammatory effects.

27. **DO:**   Astragalus herb.

Why?   It has the ability to help fight cancer in two different ways. Not only is it a huge immune system booster, it has the ability to help the immune system see cancer cells better and attack them. MD Anderson found a positive result during a study of this herb.

28. **DO:**   Use curry powder.

Why?   This extract comes from the yellow curry spice turmeric, which we already know is powerful in killing off cancerous cells in a laboratory.

29. **DO:**   Green tea is a must do. Drink it 2–4 times a day.

Why?   Green tea is known to fight cancer cells, specifically due to (EGCG), which stands for Epigallocatechin-3-gallate. That is a strong antioxidant that has been found to stop cancer cells from growing. It helps prevent new blood vessels from growing to cancerous cells.

30. **DO:** Sprinkle on some cayenne pepper.

Why? In a study with rats, it has been shown to kill cancerous tumors.

31. **DO:** Another great spice is rosemary!

Why? Rosemary has antioxidants and anti-inflammatory properties to reduce the oxidative stress that triggers many cancers. In laboratory studies, mice with skin cancer were given rosemary to reduce their development of tumors.

32. **DO:** Organic juicing or blending.

Why? The body can consume more nutrients when vegetables or fruit are ingested in a liquid form. These also help to detox the system from toxic waste. Juicing plays a huge role in detoxing the body from cancer cells.

33. **DO:** Spice things up with some dill.

Why? It has cancer preventative effects. Dill triggers the secretion of glutathione to relieve oxidative stress caused by environmental pollution. It helps prevent damaged DNA from triggering cancer.

34. **DO:** Another great herb to use is Cat's Claw.

Why? Since its use in the treatment of skin cancer, Cat's Claw has shown to visibly reduce the size of tumors. For this reason, it has gained a lot of press in recent years, even in the absence of any endorsements from the medical community.

35. **DO:** Drink lemon water in the morning, when you first wake up.

Why? If you do this 1st thing in the morning it detoxes the body and flushes out the toxins that the body discharged overnight. Also, it helps in balancing the PH.

36. **DO:** Coffee enemas. However, you must read about how to do this properly at puregirlina-toxicworld.com, or you can find it in the Gerson therapy handbook.

Why? There are so many reasons to do this; I cannot even list them all. Just to name a few:

- It helps helps detox the liver and keeps it healthy. A strong, healthy liver can aid in fighting off cancer.

- It stimulates your body to make glutathione.

- It relieves pain and inflammation in the body.

37. **DO:** Epsom salt baths, wet sauna, and dry sauna.

Why? They help to draw out toxins from the body. Remember, having a lot of toxins in the body can cause cancer.

38. **DO:** Eat cruciferous vegetables.

Why? The National Cancer Institute says that the nutrients found in vegetables like broccoli, brussel sprouts, cabbage, cauliflower, bok choy, collard greens, and arugula may lower the risk of some cancers; according to many studies from around the world.

39. **DO:** Eat berries like strawberries, blueberries, goji berries, and blackberries.

Why? These are some of the top antioxidant foods in the world. They are also high in Vitamin C which increases immune function.

40. DO: Eat citrus fruits and vegetables, such as oranges, grapefruit, carrots, squash, lemons, and sweet potatoes. (Ask your doctor, because grapefruit has the ability to make your medication stronger)

Why? Brightly colored pigments found in plant-based foods are a known sign that they are flourishing with phytonutrients; especially the carotenoids antioxidant. This is exactly the reason you should eat a variety of colored fruits and vegetables.

41. DO: Use essential oils. Lavender, frankincense, peppermint, citrus oil and spearmint are just a few examples.

Why? They help by calming you, reducing anxiety, nausea, vomiting and aiding in sleep. This can be helpful for people undergoing chemotherapy. There are many studies going on at this time for treatment with tumors. Since these are very early stages of the studies, there are no peer reviews at this time.

42. DO: Eat organic pumpkin seeds. They also make a great snack!

Why?   Believe it or not, pumpkin seeds have been linked to decreasing the risk of stomach lung, breast, prostate, and colon cancer.

43. **DO:**   Probiotics at night before you go to bed.

Why?   Probiotics are live bacteria and yeast for your immune system. They are called '*good bacteria*' to keep your gut healthy. If taken at night, your body has a chance to use more of it to build a good digestive system.

44. **DO:**   Buy PH strips and check your PH balance.

Why?   Some say disease and disorders cannot take root in a body that is PH balanced. A PH lower than 7 is said to be acidic and a PH greater than 7 is alkaline. Take a urine sample first thing in the morning and dip it onto the PH strip to get your PH balance. If you have low PH, eat more vegetables as they will alkaline your system.

45. **DO:**   Eat gluten-free.

Why?   Even if you're not gluten intolerant, gluten can cause a lot of sensitivity in some people. Many doctors say that gluten causes inflammation in humans.

Inflammation is a pre-cursor for cancer. The protiens in wheat are gut irritants.

46. **DO:** Practice meditation every day.

Why? Many studies show it can help improve sleep, focus, mood, and mental clarity, while lessening hot flashes and pain. It helps in reducing stress and boosts immune function, which is needed to fight off cancer.

47. **DO:** Practice massage, yoga, and acupuncture.

Why? All three of these reduce stress, anxiety, and pain, while lessening nausea, improving sleep, and helping to detox tissues. They also relax the body and mind.

48. **DO:** Get 7–8 hours of sleep at night.

Why? Researchers found that lack of sleep increases inflammation and disturbs normal immune function. These may promote cancer to develop in the body. If you have trouble sleeping, don't hesitate to ask your doctor for some help. Not sleeping well when diagnosed with cancer is normal, but sometimes it can be more harmful not to sleep.

49. DO: Treat yourself to dark chocolate 85% or higher.

Why? Yes, I said "DO" chocolate! A little each day, like a quarter of a bar or piece has a lot of antoxidants in it; which means that they may reduce cell damage.

50. DO: Exercise, if possible, outside.

Why? Regular physical activity is good for overall health. It helps reduce the risk of breast, colon, rectum, and many other cancers. The sun gives off natural Vitamin D. There is a link between low Vitamin D levels and cancer. Do both of these and you have a double dose of goodness.

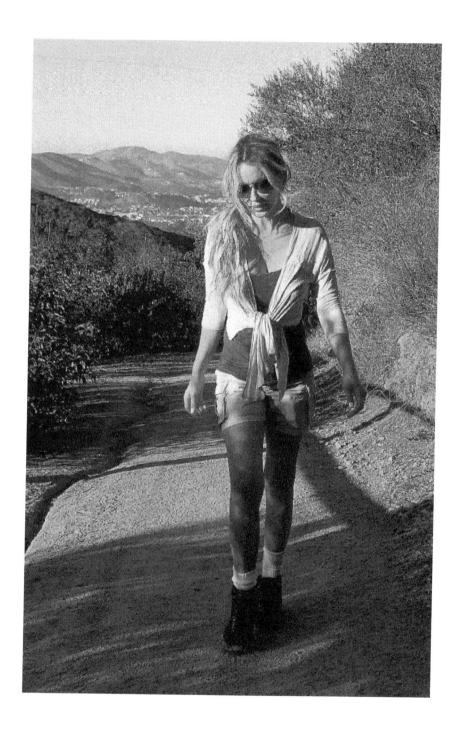

Chapter Five

Don'ts

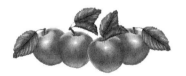

Now that I have shared with you all of the "Do's" that I recommend to many of my readers and clients, I will tell you that it was tough to narrow down both of the lists of 'Do's' and 'Don'ts'. There were so many more valuable tips that were excluded. Remember, I wanted to keep this book short and simple for people to read easily. However, you can always find more tips, do's and don'ts on my website: puregirlinatoxicworld.com, as well as Facebook and Instagram. I want to reach – and help – as many people as I can.

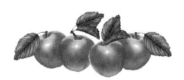

1. **DON'T:**   Make any huge decisions right now.

    Why?   You are the number one priority. Having cancer is already an emotional overload; therefore, it is not a good time to make big decisions.

2. DON'T: Don't eat sugar.

Why? Cancer cells feed off glucose, which is sugar. You don't need to add any extra sugar for cancer cells to grow.

3. DON'T: Stop eating dairy! Yes, that's what I said, no cheese, milk, yogurt, etc.

Why? Besides sugar, the second biggest thing cancer cells need to multiply is mucus. Eating dairy products create mucus in the body.

4. DON'T: Smoke, or be around secondhand smoke.

Why? It's CARCINOGENIC, which leads to cancer. Cigarettes have over 4,000 chemicals, including 43 known CARCINOGENICS and 400+ other toxins.

5. DON'T: Do not eat processed food. Stop now, *please.*

Why? Processed foods have a lot of hidden sugars, preservatives, chemicals, artificial flavors, colorings, and additives that are linked to cancer.

6. DON'T: Do not use any pesticide or herbicides on your property.

Why? They have toxic chemicals and toxins that are linked to cancer. That's why I recommend eating all-organic.

7. DON'T: Don't eat genetically modified food. No GMO's.

Why? The food is not in its pure state. The body does not recognize it as real food. GMO's can leave materials behind inside the body for a very long time. They also contain higher residues of toxic herbicide, which is linked to cancer. Point being; GMO's are CARCINOGENIC.

8. DON'T: Don't consume artificial sweeteners.

Why? It can destroy your gut flora up to 50% and the gut makes up for about 70% of your immune system. Also, when heated, artificial sweeteners fall into an extremely dangerous class of CARCINOGENIC called Dioxin, causing inflammation in the body.

9. DON'T: Use any toxic materials in your home. No paints, glues, new flooring, or toxic products.

Why? These are loaded with chemicals. If you are remodeling, make sure to use low chemicals and stay away from the home until everything dries.

10. **DON'T:** Use toxic hair dyes.

Why? They get into the bloodstream through the pores of your scalp. Hair dyes have carcinogics in them called formaldehyde. Go to puregirlinatoxicworld.com to find organic healthier hair dyes.

11. **DON'T:** Drink from plastic water bottles. It's best not to keep your food in plastic either.

Why? It has BPA in it, which is a chemical found in plastic bottles, containers, cups, and disposable plates, etc. Research strongly suggests that BPA may cause cancer in people. Especially in women – this chemical acts like a synthetic estrogen – throwing off normal hormone functions. Plastic is more toxic when frozen or heated. It lets off gasses into liquid or solid foods. Look for the BPA-free symbol, which means it does not have the chemical in it.

12. **DON'T:** Cook food in plastic containers in the microwave.

Why? As stated above, heating or freezing plastic emits gasses into your food or beverages.

13. **DON'T:** Use nail polish.

Why? Nail polishes have a lot of chemicals in them. They contain formaldehyde, which as previously mentioned, has been classified as a CARCINOGENIC. Visit puregirlinatoxicworld.com to find non-cancer causing nail polishes.

14. **DON'T:** Don't go to nail salons or hair salons without wearing a mask.

Why? There are harmful chemicals used in these places, which are known CARCINOGENICS. Try to find organic salons in your area, or one with good ventilation. Bring your own organic nail polish.

15. **DON'T:** Don't use acrylic nails.

Why? Chemicals and glues that are harmful to the body and compromise the immune system can be found in acrylic nails. Go to puregirlinatoxicworld's website to find healthy alternatives.

16. **DON'T:** Drink alcohol.

Why? Research has linked multiple ways alcohol can increase the risk of cancer. Including metabolizing ethanol in alcohol drinks to acetaldehyde, which is a toxic chemical and a human CARCINOGENIC. Acetaldehyde can damage both DNA and proteins. Alcohol also damages the liver and has been linked to liver, colon, breast, and rectum cancer. Plus, it turns into pure sugar in your system, and we already know what that does to cancer cells. So, this is a double no-no. Once you're through with your treatment or cancer-free, this is not to say that you can't have an occasional drink (but don't forget to refer to #36 in the do's within 24 hours thereafter).

17. **DON'T:** Use aluminum or products that have aluminum in them.

Why? Products that have aluminum are known as a CARCINOGENIC and may be linked to some cancers.

18. **DON'T:** Use sun tanning beds or sun lamps, and don't stay out in the sun too long without adequate protection.

Why? Too much UV radiation can cause skin cancer.

19. **DON'T:** Don't drink regular tap water.

Why? Tap water is treated with a large number of chemicals in order to kill bacteria and other microorganisms. Over 300 chemicals can be found in tap water, as well as prescription drugs and hormones. These chemicals get trapped in our cells, which then become toxic.

20. **DON'T:** Do not work in a field, factory, or company that exposes you to a wide variety of chemicals.

Why? Because chemicals can compromise the immune system and cause cancer. It's up to you to be your own advocate. If you think your work environment is unhealthy, speak up and ask what they are using and how much?

21. **DON'T:** Use talcum powder.

Why? In it's true form, some talc contains asbestos, a substance known to cause lung cancer when inhaled and ovarian cancer when used in the genital areas. Check your makeup, ladies. To find healthy, non-cancerous powders, go to puregirlinatoxicworld.com.

22. **DON'T:** Don't eat any canned foods.

Why? PFA is a chemical that seeps into the food or water in the can. This chemical has been linked to different cancers. There are cans now that are labeled PFA-free. If the can does not say that, don't buy it.

23. **DON'T:** Do not eat microwave popcorn.

Why? Microwave popcorn bags are lined with a chemical called PFOA that is known to be a CARCINOGENIC. It can cause thyroid issues, high cholesterol, bladder cancer, and pancreatic cancer.

24. **DON'T:** Do not use over-the-counter drugs unless absolutely necessary.

Why? Just like regular prescription drugs, over-the-counter drugs are toxic to the system. I am not recommending that you get off any prescription drugs. This is a conversation that you must have with your doctor.

25. **DON'T:** Don't eat animal protein.

Why? The more animal protein you eat, the more cancer you have. New, groundbreaking studies show that vegan blood is 8xs more protective against cancer cells. There are loads of research connecting animal protein intake to cancer.

26. **DON'T:** Don't eat processed meat; such as hot dogs, bacon, or deli meats.

Why? The World Health Organization says there are studies that reveal these meats are highly CARCINOGENIC. By now you know that CARCINOGENIC = cancer causing.

27. **DON'T:** Don't eat farm-raised salmon or any other farmed fish.

Why? The fish are fed chemicals, antibiotics, pesticides and other CARCINOGENICS found in materials like asbestos.

28. **DON'T:** Eat anything with white flour.

Why? White flour has a chemical called potassium bromate – a.k.a. brominated flour. This stuff helps add bulk and whiten the color of the bread. However, it is linked as a potential human carcinogen by a number of health organizations.

29. **DON'T:** Don't go in swimming pools or jacuzzis.

Why? They use a load of different chemicals. One in particular is called chlorine, which investigators found to be toxic to the body according to a study published in 2010 by The Journal of Environmental Health Preservation.

30. **DON'T:** Tap off your gas tank.

Why? The last pump of gas into your car after the nozzle clicks off does spill fuel. The vapors spoil the pump's vapor recovery function, which is designed to keep toxic chemicals out of the atmosphere. One such cancer-causing carcinogen known as benzene can get on your skin and into your lungs.

31. **DON'T:** Don't eat grilled meat.

Why? Charred and well-done meat can contain cancer elements known as hetero-cyclicamine. This happens when meat is seared at high temperatures, making it a CARCINOGENIC.

32. **DON'T:** Dry clean your clothes.

Why? According to the EPA, a solvent known as perchloroethylene is a chemical used in dry cleaning and may cause liver, kidney cancer and leukemia. Try to find organic dry cleaners near you.

33. **DON'T:** Use air fresheners, scented candles, or aerosol sprays.

Why? These products use a substance that reacts to the ozone gases. When this happens, the fragrant molecules called limonene and pinene create formaldehye. This is a known CARCINOGENIC that causes cancer.

34. **DON'T:** Do hormones unless first cleared by your doctor. This is very controversial.

Why? There are many studies that are 'pro' hormone therapy, and many studies that are against hormone therapy. However, the theory can be summed down to: "hormones are fine if there is no cancer presenting itself in the body". But if you have cancer or if there's any hereditary genes, then taking hormones is like putting gasoline on the fire. In other words, they make cancer grow.

35. **DON'T:** Use fragrances, colognes or perfumes.

Why? Some cancer prevention studies say products that have fragrance, perfume, phthalates, DEP, DBP, or DEHP as ingredients have been linked to cancer. Furthermore, it is perfectly legal for companies to use these ingredients.

Go to puregirlinatoxicworld.com to find organic alternatives.

36. **DON'T:** Forget to check all personal care, hair, and skincare products for fragrances and harmful chemicals.

Why? There are a lot of hidden fragrances disguised under different ingredients. This is also true for toxic chemicals.

Go to puregirlinatoxicworld.com to find organic replacements.

37. **DON'T:** Use art supplies and felt markers.

Why? A lot of glues, acrylic paints and solvents are used in making these pens. They have toxic chemicals in them that may be linked to cancer.

38. **DON'T:** Use deodorants or antiperspirants.

Why? These products contain a cancer causing chemical known as aluminum chlorohydrate. They go directly into the blood stream, causing the immune system to be compromised.

39. **DON'T:** Use tartar control toothpaste or ones with fluoride.

   Why? It contains preservatives and chemicals, which are known to be CARCINOGENIC. Fluoride toothpaste has chemicals in it and each chemical you put in the body can be detrimental.

40. **DON'T:** Don't use dog or cat flea collars.

   Why? They contain known neurotoxins and CARCINOGENIC compounds called propoxur. These are not only dangerous to you, but to your kids and pet, as well.

41. **DON'T:** Ladies, don't use toxic face makeup.

   Why? There are more than 80,000 chemicals used in beauty products. The FDA says that using words like *natural, non-toxic, clean* and *safe* have absolutely no official or legal meaning when it comes to cosmetics. There are loads of cancer-causing chemicals in makeup. Go to the puregirlinatoxicworld.com website to find healthier, non-cancer causing makeup alternatives.

42. **DON'T:** Hold cell phones up to your head. Do *'hands free'*.

Why? There may be evidence that cell phone use may increase the risk of brain cancer.

43. **DON'T:** Forget to check your vitamins for vitamin B.

Why? In some studies, the synthetic form of vitamin B has been linked to an increased risk of lung and prostate cancer.

44. **DON'T:** Keep yourself chronically on the go. It can cause adrenal fatigue.

Why? It's time to take care of yourself now. Slow down and breathe. Deep breathing is very healing. It brings a lots of oxygen to the cells. Cancer hates oxygen. There are some studies that state stress produces certain hormones that can make cancer tumors spread. Stress also depletes the immune system, thereby making it harder to fight cancer cells off.

45. **DON'T:** Do any unnecessary body scans.

Why? This is definitely important if you have multiple doctors. Don't be afraid to ask your doctor if the scan is really necessary. Share with all of your doctors what you're going through. Scans deliver radiation through the body, and you don't need any extra radiation. If possible, ask if you can have an MRI or ultrasound.

46. **DON'T:** Drink soda, diet soda or energy drinks! This is a biggie.

Why? Sodas and common energy drinks are filled with high amounts of sugar, dyes, and a host of many other chemicals.

47. **DON'T:** Listen to negative people or negative stories about people dying of cancer.

Why? You need to surround yourself with hope, strength, positivity, and optimistic people. Seek out cancer survivors. There are a lot of them out there. When the negative thoughts come, write them down, or call a safe person to talk to about how you're feeling. Remember, there are tons of Stage 4 and even Stage 5 cancer survivors out there. Personally, I posted pictures around my house of when I was vibrant (such as running a 5K race) and visualized getting back to that place.

48. **DON'T:** Forget to get support.

Why? You may need someone to take over your workload, help with cooking and/or caring for the children. Look into joining a cancer support group. Seek out a professional, compassionate therapist.

49. **DON'T:** Do not use toxic laundry detergent or dryer sheets.

Why? They are loaded with chemicals and CARCINOGENICS, which get on your skin, in your lungs, and then into your blood stream. Some of these have been linked to cancer. Go to puregirlinatoxicworld.com to find *'no cancer'* or *'low cancer'* detergents.

50. **DON'T:** Buy a brand new car.

Why? Brand new cars are filled with toxic chemicals that cause cancer. In the state of California, there's a sticker in every car window that states: *"Some of the products used inside this car are linked to cancer."* One of the chemicals used is formaldehyde, which is sprayed all over the dashboard and more. Ever wonder why dashboards don't crack anymore?

Even if the car is just a couple years old, it may still be releasing lower amounts of harmful chemicals. On hot days, it's best to keep windows cracked. When entering the vehicle, roll down the windows and let the off-gassing leave the car. If you love that new car smell, think again. I hope after reading this, you will reconsider.

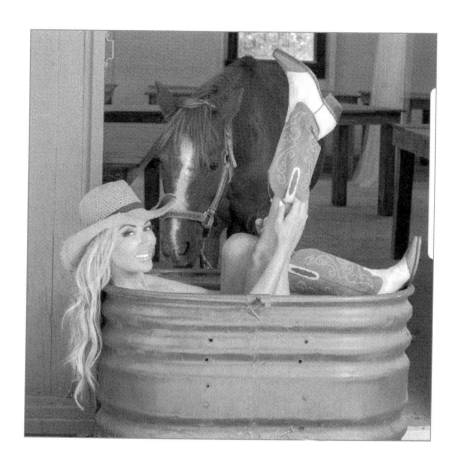

CONCLUSION

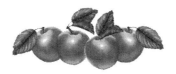

***Wow, look at you!* An official health-seeker.** You can finish your walk down health lane. However, reading about it and doing it are two different things. The power to change lies in action. You must make every effort to ensure your best chance of survival.

For those of you who are seeking cancer prevention, taking these precautions can decrease your odds of getting cancer. Remember the Sir Francis Bacon saying; *"Knowledge is power!"* This only applies if you take action.

I once read that; *"If you want your situation to change, it requires action, but if you're not willing to do the action, then your situation will not change."* So, I hope that all of my 4½ years of studying everything to do with cancer can and will help you. You now have the knowledge and now it's up to you to take the actions. I sure hope you do.

Love,

Juliet Mitchell

A.K.A. ~ *"Pure Girl in a Toxic World"*

ABOUT THE AUTHOR

JULIET MITCHELL

"What we put in our bodies is just as important as what we put on our bodies."

--- Juliet Mitchell

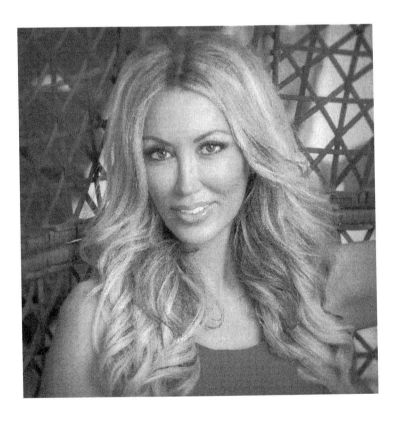

Welcome, wellness seekers!

Like you, I was searching for answers and solutions when I was diagnosed five years ago with Ovarian Cancer. I had visited my OB-GYN right before a two-week sojourn in the Sierra Mountains, and upon my return, the grim diagnosis was waiting for me. To make matters worse, the type of ovarian cancer I had – Clear Cell Carcinoma – was one of the worst, most aggressive kinds. If this was not a wakeup call, I don't know what is!

Up until that overwhelming moment, I thought I was healthy. I went to the gym five days a week and "ate right," or so I thought. But I never thought that I would not survive. God had other plans for me. My natural instinct was to get to the bottom of it and to find healing. As I went through the process of cancer treatments and chemotherapy, I soaked up any and all information. Like a sponge, I wanted to absorb everything. My thirst for knowledge was insatiable. I read books, watched documentaries, read articles, medical papers, and any literature I could find. I studied the moves of other cancer survivors to learn what they did or didn't do. However, I found it difficult to find good, clear information that was easy to digest or that wasn't over 500 pages long.

On the bright side, I discovered a common denominator between all of my research. During times of war and five years thereafter, people lived off the land and cancer rates plummeted down to zero. They ate fruits, vegetables, nuts, grains, and seeds. Hence, I quickly became a vegan. People came to me with questions, which started a "movement", per say. That is why I am here, today.

I am not a doctor, nor a nutritionist. I am a mother, daughter, fun-seeker, hiker, and golfer who is passionate about health. I'm also a blogger, video journalist, health advocate, organic living expert, public speaker, and healthy living coach. Recently, I became a member of IFOAM, Organic International, and have been a supporter and donor of the Organic Consumers Assoc. of America. I studied environmental health, nutrition, well-being and food at Harvard University.

So now, my journey led me to launch this website. I realize that what I put in my body needs to be just as pure as what I put on it. In fact, there are hardly any regulations of the 60 billion dollar a year makeup and skincare product industry. Startling, right? That's why I'm here to disclose both the toxic and non-toxic products that people commonly use. Come along with me and explore the safest, healthiest products that truly work.

TESTIMONIALS

PEOPLE I'VE HELPED

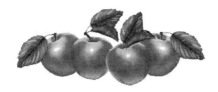

"Pure Girl has helped me reevaluate the chemicals I'm putting in my body. I don't have time or can be lazy to do much research, so I just use the brands she uses. I've changed my shampoo, toothpaste, make-up and even gum! Thank you for helping your follwers get healthier, pure girl."

-- *Edrienne Palma Baebler*

"I wanted to thank you so much for helping me see the changes that are necessary, and if we are willing to make those changes... it can truly turn our lives around and have a major impact. I have had AMAZING RESULTS! And my doctor has found NO CANCER IN MY BODY. I pray that if I continue to stick to a healthy diet, detox my liver, juice and exercise, I will live a long, healthy life. Thank you, Juliet for this valuable information!"

-- Kim Turner, R.N.

"Super knowledgeable in her field. Juliet is an inspiration!"

-- Andrew Lowen

"Juliet is America's newest rising star in the organic world. Seriously, I can't believe how much knowledge and wisdom I have learned about lifestyle, nutrition and important health topics since working with her. She has not only survived cancer and personal challenges like a Champ, she never brags about any of her awesome achievements or natural beauty. I'm really impressed by her innate passion for this niche and you should sit up and take notice! She's like a goldmine of information."

-- Anne Violette, Author, Mom of 3

"And together we will fight this!

Juliet, endless research is the magic word. It's what we want to see. Nothing less than a cancer cure, would mean so much to me and others like me...

For together we have fought this!

It'll take support from everyone, to really see this through. So peace of mind for all of us, can start off fresh and new. Reborn beginning of new is our words and spirit to be within us...

And together we will win!"

-- Mark Jones

ACKNOWLEDGEMENTS

PEOPLE WHO'VE HELPED ME

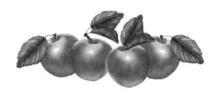

Where do I begin? Along my journey, there have been so many that I want to say thank you to or that I appreciate so much. I will start with Lisa Lennox, you were the girl that saved my life. I am so glad you told me to go to the doctor. Thank you, my guardian angel!

- A special heartfelt thanks to my family, especially my mother Helene, who sat through all of my chemotherapies with me and held me in her arms as I cried with fear of the unknown. I'll never forget the words that my mother said to me, "*I wish I could take the cancer out of your body and put it into mine. Oh God, please."* Only a mother's love could feel that way. I am so blessed to have you as my mother. I love you more than all the stars that could ever fill the universe.

- To my father John and my stepmom Brenda, thank you for being there when I woke up from surgery and for bringing me food, love, and your caring and support as I recovered from chemo. I love you so, so, so, so, so much.

- To my Stepdad Mark, thank you for your love and support through this difficult time in my life.

- To my sister Laurie and her husband, Rowdy, who came each week and brought me healthy, organic food to eat. That nourished my body as I was going through treatment. I love you.

- To my sister Jennifer – who held my hand and walked with me the first several weeks after my diagnosis and the endless phone calls of support – for you I am grateful. Thank you; I love you so very much and you know that I'm always available. Good night and God Bless.

- For my niece, Tara, who taught me all about toxic products. She took me to the store and showed me healthier options. She taught me her vegan lifestyle, of which I have adapted. I am so grateful for your love and support. I don't know if I would be here if it wasn't for you. I am eternally grateful. I love you so much.

- A heartfelt thanks to my brother Sean and to my sister Helen for all your love, prayers and support. I love you more than you'll ever know.

- With a grateful heart, I want to say thank you to Miss Mary Halls, one of my closest friends. She gave me my first wellness book and thus began my journey to good health. She was a beacon of light in my darkest hour and my cheerleader on my winning drives. I love you so much.

- A deep thank you to one of my best friends in the whole world, Miles Stanich. I love you more than you will ever know. Your relentless support, guiding direction and love in my hardest times of life is so much appreciated. Always there on the other end of the phone to tell me, *"Juliet, you're going to be okay."* I love you, my friend... always and forever.

- To my sweet Parvaneh Zargar – my other best friend in the whole world. I am so lucky to have two. Parvaneh was the beautiful woman that was there every Saturday after chemo to take care of the sick Juliet. She was cooking, cleaning, and organizing my drawers. For her endless love, support, and caring, I am so grateful. Thank you for making me laugh when I really wanted to cry. I love you, daisy girl.

- All the love to Joan, who took care of me after my chemotherapy until I was strong enough to take care of myself. I am grateful for the talks that we had about God. You gave me the strength to continue to fight. I am so thankful that God brought you into my life. I love you and you are an amazing woman.

- I am grateful to my special friend, Heidi, who came and slept each Friday night with me after I received chemo. Your love and your support during the darkest time in my life meant the world to me. I love you, Heidi girl!

- Very special thank you to Steve Vanderhei, my ex-husband, for the years after cancer. Your caring, love and support was incredible. You bought my expensive juicer for me. You helped me get on the path to health. I am so grateful for this and will always love you.

- To Annie, you are the best ghostwriter in the world. Thank you for letting me spread my word. I am grateful that God brought you into my life. Here's to another couple books, baby girl.

- To Marc Druhot, who fought the fight of cancer. He may not be with us in the human form any longer, but he's with us in spirit. He did not lose to cancer. He rose to meet the challenge and he showed up. His mission was complete and he impacted so many lives for the better. Until we meet again. Love, Juliet.

- To Mike Salazar – a father, husband, son, and friend – you were loved by many and will always be remembered.

- To all men, women, and children who have fought and are no longer with us, I tell you in spirit that you did not lose; you were a fighter! Anyone that fights cancer is not a loser.

- To Doctor Truong, who didn't skip a beat. Her relentless perfectionism as a doctor is the one that found my cancer. If it wasn't for you, I wouldn't be alive.

- To my sweet, Godly friend Robin, who I met the day that I came out of my oncologist's office. We locked eyes and were instant cancer warriors together in this fight. She walked me through my first day with chemo, who I laughed and cried with along my journey, and who helped me find a deeper relationship with God.

REFERENCES

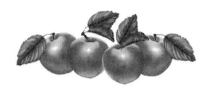

- MD Anderson. Org
- Health news. Org
- Gerson Therapy
- Integrative cancer
- Livescience.com
- Harvard University
- Mayo Clinic
- Natural Living Ideas
- Mercola.com
- Thetonic.com
- Pacific College
- China Study
- Forks Over Knives Documentary

- Mindbody.com
- University of Minnesota
- WebMD
- NBC News
- The truth about cancer
- Natural resource defense counsel
- "What The Health" Documentary
- The Huffington Post
- E.P.A Cancer Panel
- AJC.Com
- Natural Health News
- Breastcancer.org
- Immunehealthscience.com
- The American Cancer Society
- Fox News
- UnderGround Health Report
- Cancer.org
- National Cancer Institute
- EWG Skin Deep
- John Hopkins University
- Nature News.com
- One Take Nutrition

- Mind Body. Com
- Time Magazine
- The Guardian.com
- Cancer Research UK
- Cancer Treatment Center of America
- International Agency for Cancer Research

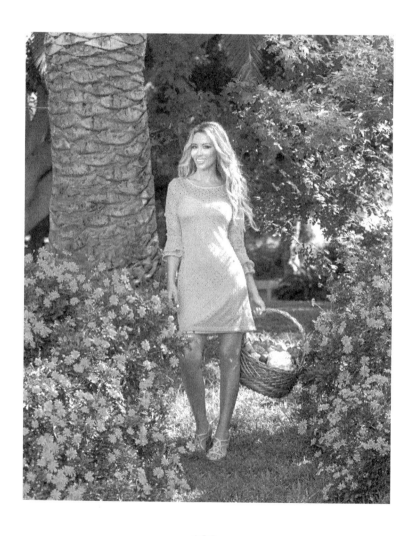

NOTE TAKING

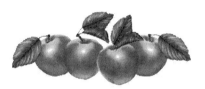

_____

_____

_____

_____

_____

_____

_____

_____

_____

_____

_____

_____

_____

_____

_____

_____

_____

_____

_____

_____

_____

_____

_____

_____

_____

_____

_____

_____

_____

_____

_____

_____

_____

_____

_____

_____

_____

_____

_____

_____

_____

_____

_____

_____

_____

_____

_____

_____

_____

_____

_____

_____

_____

_____

_____

_____

_____

_____

_____

_____

_____

_____

_____

_____

_____

_____

_____

_____

_____

_____

_____

_____

_____

_____

_____

_____

_____

_____

_____

_____

_____

_____

_____

I hope you have a remarkable journey!

There are some people that do not want to do chemotherapy or radiation, and others whose doctors have said there is nothing more that can be done to help them. For those people in search of alternative treatments, I refer the Northern Baja Gerson Center. Dr. Patrick Vicker is the best and really cares about his patients.

~ *Juliet Mitchell*

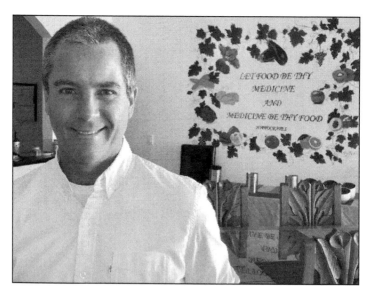

You can find out more about this alternative cancer treatment center at:

www.gersontreatment.com
Dr. Patrick Vickers
Northern Baja Gerson Center
Email: info@gersontreatment.com
715-299-5070

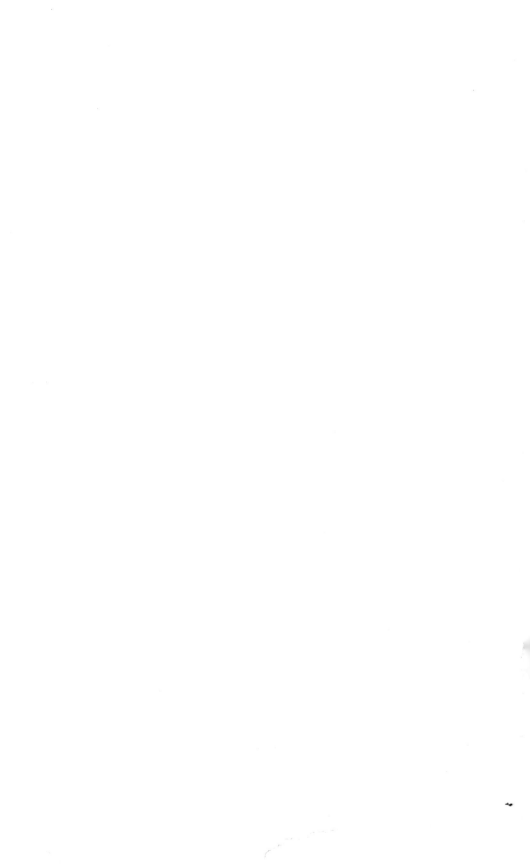

90993039R10078

Made in the USA
San Bernardino, CA
17 October 2018